COUNTRY DOCTOR'S
⊷ BOOK OF ⊶
REMEDIES
& CURES

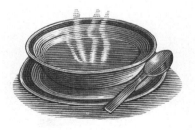

Publications International, Ltd.

Contents

❖ ❖ ❖ ❖

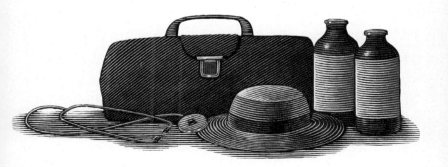

Reap the Benefits of Country Living

❖ ❖ ❖ ❖

Life is just simpler in the country. The pace is slower, the air is fresher, and the nights are clearer. Sure, we can see why some people like city life, with all its flash and noise, but for country folks, nothing is better than living close to the land and enjoying it. This unhurried life includes using simple solutions for the same health problems city folks face. Whether we're talking allergies, colds, headaches, or muscle pain, we prefer using unassuming, tried-and-true methods of relief rather than chemicals developed in a laboratory.

In *Country Doctor's Book of Remedies & Cures*, we've gathered easy strategies to deal with 24 everyday health problems. These aren't miracle cures or snake oil tonics—they're simple solutions that can be found in your kitchen, your garden, or your local store. Many require only an easy change in your behavior. Let country wisdom be the key to your improved health!

This book is designed to help you help yourself, but we encourage you to discuss these remedies with your doctor. The two of you know all about your current health status and the medications you take. If any ailment you are self-treating with the advice presented here doesn't improve or gets worse, you need to see your health-care provider right away.

Allergies

❖ ❖ ❖ ❖

Those who work outside know they're at the mercy of the environment, but for many folks, comfort has nothing to do with rain, snow, heat, or wind. For these people, common hay fever and allergies sure do make a mess of things. But staying inside isn't the answer, because plenty of allergens there cause sneezing, itching, and watery eyes, too. Instead of reaching for the antihistamines, nose sprays, and eyedrops, try these simple fixes.

Relax with a washcloth. If your sinuses are congested and making your head feel like it's hitting the business end of a bucking bronco, soak a washcloth in warm water and place it over your nose and upper-cheek area. Kick up your feet and lean your head back a bit to feel your pain float away.

Get saltwater relief. Irrigating the nose with saline solution (salt water) may help soothe upper-respiratory allergies by removing irritants that become stuck in the nose and cause inflammation. You can buy saline solution at your local drugstore, or you can make your own fresh solution daily by mixing a teaspoon of salt in a pint of warm distilled water and adding a pinch of baking soda. Bend over a sink and sniff a bit of solution into one nostril at a time,

Bust the Dust

The following tips can help you make your bedroom less hospitable to dust mites—microscopic insects that feed on your dead skin cells. The feces and corpses of these little buggers trigger allergies in millions of people. Since the bedroom is the dust mite's favorite hangout, and you spend at least a third of your life there, you need to allergy-proof it.

- Encase pillows and mattresses in airtight, plastic or vinyl cases or special covers.
- Wash your bedding in hot water every seven to ten days.
- Clean once a week.
- Avoid fabric-covered furniture.
- Vacuum the window treatments.
- Don't use the bedroom as storage space.
- Clean out your air conditioner and heating ducts.

allowing it to drain back out through the nose or mouth; do this once or twice a day. (However, if you also have asthma, check with your doctor before trying this remedy.)

Wash up. If you're out enjoying the land during pollen season, you might bring sticky yellow pollen back inside with you—all over your hair and body. If you don't wash up, chances are good that pollen will find its way into your eyes and lungs, causing your allergies to flare. Once indoors, take a hot shower and wash your hair. This will remove the pollen, and the steam will open up your sinuses.

Shut the windows. Nothing beats a fresh country breeze blowing through the house, but pollen is probably hitching a ride. Close the windows to minimize contact with the powdery stuff.

Go bare. Carpets hide dust mites, which are tiny critters whose droppings spur allergies in millions of people. Bare floors, vacuumed and damp-mopped frequently, will help keep your home's dust mite population down (you can't get rid of them all). If you can't remove all the carpeting in your home, at least opt for bare floors in the bedroom, where you spend most of your time while in the house.

Think before you burn. Many folks who live in rural areas are allowed to burn household and construction refuse, but the smoke from burning wood that has been treated with heavy metals or other chemical-laden materials can trigger awful reactions in people with allergies, asthma, or sensitive respiratory systems. Also, burn only clean, untreated material in the fireplace.

Ride horseradish to relief. Horseradish has been used in America for generations to treat hay fever. If you've eaten it, you know it can cause your eyes to water and your sinuses to burn. The cause is something called allyl isothiocyanate. Scientific studies have shown that allyl isothiocyanate has decongestant and antiasthmatic properties. Take $\frac{1}{4}$ teaspoon of condiment horseradish during a congestive hay fever attack. You can take horseradish as often as you like, but be careful, because some people have a skin allergy to it.

Arthritis

❖ ❖ ❖ ❖

According to the Arthritis Foundation, more than 46 million people in the United States are in the grip of one of 100 different kinds of arthritis. The two main forms are osteoarthritis, where the cartilage that surrounds bones breaks down, and rheumatoid arthritis, where the body's immune system attacks the lining of joints. Unfortunately, there is no cure for the painful effects of arthritis, but there are simple, down-home strategies that can make living with it easier.

Easing Stiffness

Try the following tips to lessen arthritis pain:

Get moving. Living an active life is not only good for the soul, it's also good for your joints. Your doctor can tell you what exercises are best.

Get wet. A warm pool, lake, or swimming hole will loosen your muscles and joints, and working out in the water will be easier because of the buoyancy. Ask your doctor if heated water is okay if you are pregnant or have any chronic health problems.

Put on a scarf. Wrap a scarf around the painful joints to keep them warm, just don't put it on too tightly.

Protecting Your Joints

Take the load off tender joints and save them from stressful tasks whenever you can. The following suggestions will help you safeguard your hands and wrists:

Spread the strain. You want to avoid tight grips and putting too much pressure on your fingers, so try to use the palms of your hands to pick up plates, pots, pans, and heavy tools.

"Arm" yourself. Use your arm instead of your hand whenever possible. For example, push open those heavy doors with the side of your arm instead of your outstretched hand.

Pad those handles. Look for household tools, utensils, and writing implements that have chunky, padded handles. You can also add your own padding by taping foam rubber around the handles of almost anything you grip to use.

Get loopy. Tie loops made from rope or bandannas to door handles, like those on the refrigerator and oven. You won't need as tight of a grip to open them.

Natural Relief

If nature can support so many different plants and critters, you can bet she can produce ways to help soothe arthritis discomfort. Try these tips:

A hot idea. Cayenne pepper isn't just for spicing up bland meatloaf; it's been used around the world for centuries as a counterirritant. Cayenne works as a topical pain reliever by reducing the activity of substance P, a chemical in your body that carries pain messages from the skin's nerve endings. Place one ounce of cayenne pepper in one quart of rubbing alcohol. Let stand three weeks, shaking the bottle each day. Then strain, and use a cloth to apply the liniment to affected areas. Leave it on for 10 to 20 minutes, then rinse it off.

Get sold on celery. The celery plant contains more than 25 different anti-inflammatory compounds, and it's plumb full of minerals. A cup of celery contains more than 340 milligrams of potassium, and that's important because a potassium deficiency may contribute to some arthritis symptoms. Try the following celery tea recipe: Put one teaspoon of celery seeds in a cup, and fill the cup with boiling water. Cover and let stand for 15 minutes before straining and drinking. Drink three cups a day during an acute arthritis attack.

Athlete's Foot

❖ ❖ ❖ ❖

Athlete's foot is a fungal infection of the feet that causes redness, itching, cracking, and scaling of the skin of the feet. In severe cases, blisters form on the soles; these blisters produce stinging pain and are vulnerable to secondary infection. Although it's uncomfortable for anyone, athlete's foot is downright unbearable for those who spend all day on their feet.

You'll have to see the doctor for severe or stubborn cases, but most of the time you can treat athlete's foot under your own roof. Before you buy one of those antifungal powders, lotions, or sprays, try the following:

Keep your dogs dry. Everything you do to fight athlete's foot should revolve around keeping your feet as dry as possible.

Soap up. Wash your feet twice a day with soap and water, and dry them thoroughly; pay special attention to the skin between your toes.

Make tea for toes. To help dry out the infection and ease the itching, steep six black tea bags in a quart of warm water and soak your feet in it. The tannins in the tea may do the trick.

Don't bleach. Home remedies that involve strong chemicals and solvents, such as bleach, alcohol, or floor cleaners, are as bad an idea as planting corn in February. These products can severely damage your skin.

Treat your shoes. If you've got a fungus on your feet, you've also got a fungus in your footwear. Treat the inside of your shoes or your boots with Lysol spray every time you take them off.

Air 'em out. Those sunny days aren't just good for hitting the swimming hole, they're also great for your shoes. Take the laces out, pull up their tongues, and set your shoes outside in a sunny, well-ventilated place. The sunshine and circulating air will help dry out the shoes and kill the fungus.

"Aloe" for some plant help. Although the juice of the aloe vera plant is best known for its ability to treat burns, it also holds its own against athlete's foot fungus. Scientists have found that aloe vera juice not only promotes the growth of healthy tissue, it also acts as a disinfectant.

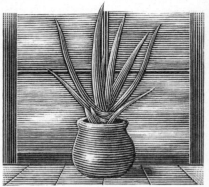

Break off a part of the aloe vera leaf and apply the juicy sap to the infected area. If you don't want to grow your own aloe vera plant, you can buy aloe vera gel at your local drugstore.

Go with garlic and vinegar. Certain cooking staples can double as effective medications. Just like a barn cat chases off mice, garlic is extremely inhospitable to tiny intruders, in this case, fungi and bacteria. Try soaking your feet once a day in a garlic footbath. Blend two whole garlic bulbs in a blender, and add to a quart of hot water. Fill a small tub with enough hot water to cover your feet, then add the garlic water. Soak for 20 minutes, then dry thoroughly.

The Amish have a similar cure that uses vinegar. Mix one cup of vinegar with two quarts of water and soak your feet in it every night for 15 to 30 minutes (use a fresh bath every night). Or you can mix a cup of vinegar with a cup of water and apply the solution to your feet with a cotton ball. Make sure your feet are completely dry before putting on your socks and shoes. Like garlic, vinegar is tough on microscopic critters.

Back Pain

❖ ❖ ❖ ❖

Country folks know hard work is hard on the back. For many, being close to the land sometimes makes them feel like they're the ones holding up the earth. No matter how many times "lift with your legs, not your back" has been said, the back still ends up taking the brunt. Aspirin, ibuprofen, and acetaminophen are safe pain relievers (but never give aspirin to anyone younger than 18 unless under doctor's orders because of the threat of Reye's syndrome, and pregnant women should ask their doctors before taking anything); however, there are more natural ways to ease the pain.

Don't take it lying down. You'll want to get moving as soon as possible because lying around like a hound dog in August may make your pain worse. At the least, it doesn't appear to speed up recovery. If you feel you must rest it, lie flat on your back with two pillows underneath your knees. And don't rest or sleep on your stomach for long periods; you may hurt your neck because you have to twist it just to breathe. Try to get up and move around—slowly and gently—as soon as possible. Any more than three days of bed rest could weaken the muscles and make them more prone to strain.

Ice it. Get ice on the painful area within 24 hours of a strain. Ice keeps tissue inflammation to a minimum and eases discomfort by decreasing the ability of nerves to send pain signals to the brain (think molasses in January). Place ice cubes in a plastic bag, then place the bag on top of a thin towel that covers the skin. Leave the ice pack on for 20 minutes, take it off for 30 minutes, and then replace it for another 20 minutes.

Take a hot bath. If it's been more than a day since you wrenched your back, ice won't help. Instead, try soaking in a tub of hot water for 20 minutes or more to loosen the muscles. Pregnant women, however, should not sit in a hot bath or hot tub for too long, because raising the body temperature over 100 degrees Fahrenheit for long periods may cause birth defects or miscarriage (contact your doctor first to find out if a soak is okay).

Relax. Emotional stress causes a lot of back pain. Learn and practice a relaxation technique, such as a deep-breathing exercise. Head out to the porch, close your eyes, and breathe slowly and deeply, counting backward from 100. If you aren't lucky enough to live in the quiet country, try picturing yourself there to help yourself relax.

Prevent the Pain

Any mechanic will tell you it's easier to properly maintain equipment than to fix something that breaks. The same is true with your back. Try these tips to avoid having your back go out in the first place.

Cushion your ride. Many car and truck seats aren't designed to support the small of your back. If yours doesn't, use a small cushion or rolled-up towel to provide the missing support. And on long drives, get out and stretch every couple hours to increase blood flow and decrease stiffness.

Carry objects close to your body. When picking up and carrying something heavy, pull in your elbows and hold the object close to your body. When reaching up for a bulky item, stand beneath it and rest it on your head. That way your spine, not your back muscles, carries the weight.

Drop excess baggage. Maintaining a healthful body weight helps lighten your back's load. What's more, having a flabby midsection may cause you to become sway-backed, which can worsen back pain.

Blisters

❖ ❖ ❖ ❖

"**B**lister" might as well be a four-letter word to anyone who started the day with one and then had to gut out 8, 10, or 12 hours on his or her feet. These tender spots that fill up with fluid (released by tiny blood vessels in an area where delicate skin tissues have been burned, pinched, or just plain irritated) may be the enemy most hated by the working man and working woman. Virtually everyone has experienced friction blisters, those varmints caused by hot, sweaty feet and/or ill-fitting shoes or boots. Read on to find out how you can get back on your feet.

Pitch a tent. No, you're not heading into the woods for a little fishing; you're "tenting" the adhesive bandage you're using to cover your blister. Instead of placing the bandage right on top of the blister, bring in the bandage's sides so the padding in the middle of the bandage raises up a bit. Securing the bandage this way protects the tender area but still exposes it to air, which will speed healing.

Let it breathe. Some doctors say you need to give your blistered foot the dog-in-a-car treatment: expose it to as much air as possible. You probably won't drive down the road with your foot sticking out of the window, but you may want to go without the bandage occasionally.

Pad it. When you have a blister on the bottom of your foot, you might need more padding than a regular bandage gives you. Look in the foot-care aisle of your drugstore for circular foam pads, or ask the pharmacist for sheets of padding. You can use either to surround your your blister with a protective foam donut. Then cover the blister with some antibacterial ointment, and put a bandage over the whole shebang.

Put it up. Elevating the blistered area can help relieve pressure and ease pain.

Drain it. Because of the risk of infection, popping a blister shouldn't be your first option, but a blister causing extreme pressure—such as one on a finger or toe or under a nail—is a candidate for draining. However, you should never open a blister caused by a burn. A doctor should also treat large blisters that may open on their own due to friction.

If you choose to pop it, wipe the blister and a sewing needle with rubbing alcohol. Prick the blister once or twice near its edge, then slowly and gently press out the fluid. Leave the deflated skin covering of the blister in place; it is called the blister's roof, and it protects the wound from infection and acts as a bridge for healing cells. Finally, apply antibacterial ointment to the blister, and cover with a bandage.

Colds

❖ ❖ ❖ ❖

Just as sure as you know the sun will rise in the east and set in the west, you can bet a cold will somehow affect you this year. Why are colds as seemingly unstoppable as mosquitoes at the lake? More than 200 different kinds of viruses cause the upper-respiratory infection known as the common cold, and these viruses easily jump from person to person, so the sneezing, stuffy nose, cough, sore throat, headache, and touch of fever get spun around the population like square dancers.

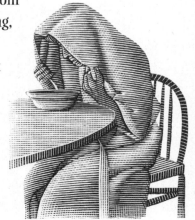

And there isn't much you can do about it. Despite the billions of dollars spent every year on medicines, there is no cure for the common cold. As the saying goes: "Do nothing and your cold will last seven days. Do everything and it will last a week." The symptoms you experience as a cold are actually parts of the body's natural immune response. In fact, by the time you feel you're coming down with a cold, you've likely been infected for a day and a half. Following simple self-care techniques may help you feel more comfortable and help your body heal itself as quickly as possible.

Drink plenty of fluids. Fluids may help thin the mucus, thus keeping it flowing freely and helping the body to expel it—along with the viral particles that get trapped in it. Water and other liquids also combat dehydration. Drink at least eight ounces of fluid every two hours.

Follow Mom's advice. It turns out chicken soup is good for the body as well as the soul, especially if the body is fighting a cold. There are several theories about why chicken soup helps. It's a liquid, so it helps prevent dehydration, and it thins mucous secretions. It's also hot, which may promote blood circulation in the throat, and that blood carries the body's natural cold-fighters. The soup's steamy vapors may also help to open clogged sinuses. And if you add some naturally antimicrobial garlic to the recipe, you may have yourself a killer cold fighter, and a tasty one at that.

Rest. Working when you have a cold will leave you exhausted, and it will put your coworkers at risk of catching your infection. So do everyone a favor and stay home.

Gargle with warm salt water. It may not taste great, but gargling with warm salt water ($\frac{1}{4}$ teaspoon salt in four ounces warm water) every one to two hours can soothe a sore, scratchy throat. Salt water is an astringent (meaning it causes tissue to contract), which can soothe inflammation in the throat and may help loosen mucus.

Use a saltwater wash. The body makes infection-fighting molecules called cytokines, or lymphokines, which do a pretty decent job, but they cause inflammation and swelling in the nose. Washing away these molecules with salt water can reduce nasal swelling. Mix one level teaspoon salt in one quart water and fill a clean nasal-spray bottle with the mixture (save the leftover solution for later). Spray the salt water three or four times into each nostril. Repeat five to six times per day.

Drink ginger tea. Ginger tea is a traditional cold remedy in several regions of the United States. Ginger induces sweating, which helps to cool the body during fever, and it contains 12 different aromatic anti-inflammatory compounds, including some with aspirinlike effects.

Cut a fresh gingerroot into thin slices and place in a pot with one quart of water. Bring to a boil, then cover the pot and simmer on the lowest possible heat for 30 minutes. Let cool for 30 minutes more before straining. Drink $\frac{1}{2}$ to one cup three to five times a day. Sweeten with honey, as desired (but never give honey to a child younger than two).

Vaporize it. Dry nasal membranes don't work as well to foil viral invasions, so plug in a humidifier to moisten your environment and keep your nasal tissues moist (and comfortable). If you don't have a humidifier, you can drape a towel over your head and bend over a pot of steaming-hot water; just be careful not to burn yourself.

Constipation

❖ ❖ ❖ ❖

Irregularity is one of those topics that isn't brought up at the dinner table—or anywhere else, for that matter. Bowel habits are very personal, and changes in them that cause problems, such as constipation, can be embarrassing. But regularity is a relative term: for some people, it means three bowel movements per day; for others, it means three per week. Any sudden change in bowel habits, however, requires a doctor visit to rule out serious problems. For the occasional bout with constipation, there are some simple tips that can get you back on schedule.

Get moving. When you're moving, so are your bowels, and if you spend most of your time sitting around, your bowels will be sluggish. You don't have to run a marathon or bale hay for eight hours; just get out for a nice stroll every day.

Raise your glass. Keeping your body hydrated can relieve constipation or keep it from happening in the first place.

Farmers know crops can't push up through a dry field, so they irrigate. Similarly, your stool becomes dry and difficult to pass when you're dehydrated. Try to drink eight cups of fluid throughout the day, and make most of that water.

Find some fiber.
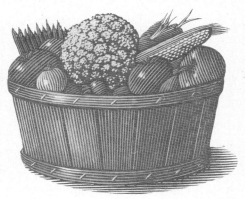
Farmers also know that to get something good out, you have to put good stuff in. When it comes to your body, you need to put fiber in to get your stool out. Fiber is the indigestible part of plant foods. It adds mass to the stool and helps the colon push things along. Avoid or remedy constipation by gradually raising your daily fiber intake to 20 to 35 grams. You'll get the most fiber from fresh and minimally processed fruits, vegetables, grains, and beans.

Say yes to sesame seeds. The Amish, who live closer to the land than anyone in North America, use sesame seeds as a laxative. The seeds are nutritious and contain about 55 percent oil, which helps to lubricate the intestines. Try eating as much as $\frac{1}{2}$ ounce of sesame seeds a day to get relief. An easy way to do it is to grind fresh seeds in a coffee grinder and sprinkle them on food like a condiment.

Serve some Epsom. Epsom salts act as a laxative by drawing water into the intestines, which helps ease out the stool.

Mix two or three teaspoons of Epsom salts in a glass of warm water and drink. Do this once a day, but not for more than seven days. Habitual use of Epsom salts can cause dehydration and laxative dependence.

Diarrhea

❖ ❖ ❖ ❖

If you're saddled with a case of diarrhea, you're probably not trotting far from the homestead. Although it's uncomfortable and unpleasant, diarrhea is generally like a garter snake: quick moving, but with a harmless bite. And unless diarrhea persists for more than two or three days (a sign you should see the doctor), you usually don't find out what caused it. What's important to remember about diarrhea is that your body is trying to get rid of something that is bad, so, in most cases, you shouldn't try to stop it with antidiarrheal tablets or liquids. Your best bet is to try these coping tips.

Keep hydrated. Dehydration is the most serious consequence of diarrhea, so you want to keep drinking to stay hydrated. But your body also loses electrolytes during a case of the trots. Electrolytes are minerals like sodium and potassium that help run body processes, so you'll want to replace these during a prolonged case of diarrhea. Aim for sipping (don't gulp) eight cups of cool (not ice-cold)

Hello, Doc?

Most cases of diarrhea aren't serious, but you should see your doctor if:

❖ there is blood in the stool.

❖ you experience symptoms of dehydration (dizziness, deep-yellow urine, increased thirst, or dry skin; children may also cry without producing tears).

❖ you have a fever or shaking chills.

❖ your diarrhea persists for more than two to three days.

❖ the person who has diarrhea is very young, very old, or has a chronic health condition.

---

fluids per day, twelve if you also have a fever. Water; weak tea with a little sugar; sports drinks, such as Gatorade; flat soda pop (decaffeinated flavors like ginger ale are best); and fruit juices, other than apple and prune (which have a laxative effect), are all good choices. You can also try electrolyte-replacement formulas, such as Pedialyte, Rehydralyte, or Ricelyte, available at drugstores.

Eat easy-to-digest foods. Soup, gelatin, rice, plain noodles, bananas, potatoes, toast, soda crackers, and skinless white-meat chicken are all safe. Avoid dairy products (except yogurt that has gut-friendly live lactobacillus cultures) and greasy or sugary foods.

Cut the caffeine. Caffeine stimulates your entire body, including your intestines, and you want that right now as much as you want flies at your barbecue.

Warm the belly. Putting a heating pad or hot-water bottle on your stomach may help with abdominal cramps.

Try some herbs. Chamomile has long been used to treat tummy troubles because the herb contains strong anti-inflammatory oils and other active ingredients, and it has antispasmodic properties. Those who use it recommend adding peppermint to increase its effectiveness. Put one teaspoon of chamomile flowers and one teaspoon of peppermint leaves in a cup, and fill the cup with boiling water. Let that steep, covered, for 15 minutes before straining and drinking. Sip three cups per day.

Flu

❖ ❖ ❖ ❖

When it comes to illnesses, the flu is like a tornado, flood, and fire rolled into one heaping mess of trouble. No other sickness seems to cut as wide a swath as the flu—when one person gets this respiratory infection, it seems as though everyone soon has it.

The flu's symptoms are similar to the common cold, but it is much more serious. Influenza causes high fever, sore throat, dry cough, severe muscle aches and pains, fatigue, loss of appetite, and pain and stiffness in the joints. But unlike the common cold, the flu kills about 36,000 Americans every year, according to the Centers for Disease Control and Prevention. What makes the flu tough to track and kill is the fact that there are different strains of the virus, and the strain that causes most of the damage changes annually. Researchers have to predict which strain will be the major one in order to create enough effective vaccine; if they're wrong, more people will be infected that year.

It sounds like fishing without knowing what kind of bait to use, but if you do happen to get caught by the flu, there are ways to ease some of the discomfort and help your body fight back without resorting to over-the-counter or prescription medications.

Get plenty of rest. Plan on sleeping and otherwise taking it easy for a few days. This shouldn't be hard to do considering fatigue is one of the main symptoms.

Make it a fluid situation. Drinking plenty of any nonalcoholic, decaffeinated liquid will help keep you hydrated and will also thin mucous secretions. (Booze and caffeine make your body lose fluid.) If you're not eating, juice can help supply some of the nutrients usually provided by food.

Humidify. The influenza virus loves dry air, and the artificial heat your furnace pumps out lowers your home's humidity level. Using a humidifier may not only help prevent the spread of the flu but may also make you feel more comfortable if you do get it.

Encourage a good cough. If your cough is producing mucus, that's a good thing, so don't take medicines to suppress it. Drinking fluids will help bring up the mucus of a productive cough and will ease the cough a bit, too.

Make thyme. One helper that comes from the kitchen is thyme. Hot thyme tea makes you sweat, which helps cool a fever. Plus, thyme contains thymol, which is a powerful expectorant and antiseptic. Thymol disperses in the steam of a hot tea, so inhaling the steam can spread the thymol throughout the mucous membranes of the upper-respiratory tract like gossip through a quilting bee. Once it gets around, thymol may help keep bacteria, viruses, and fungi from infecting body membranes. Thyme also has mild analgesic and fever-reducing properties.

Put one teaspoon of dried thyme leaves in a cup, and fill the cup with boiling water. Let steep for five minutes while inhaling the steam through your nose and mouth. Then, strain the tea, sweeten with honey (but never give honey to a child younger than two), and sip slowly.

Get lemon aid. If viruses and bacteria are the Hatfields, lemon juice is a McCoy—they just don't get along with each other. Drinking hot lemonade creates an environment inhospitable to the bugs, so the tart tonic might work against the flu. Plus, lemon rind is full of lemon oil, which has antibacterial, antiviral, antifungal, and anti-inflammatory constituents. Five of these specifically battle influenza viruses. Lemon oil is also an expectorant.

Chop one whole lemon and put it, peel and all, in a pot. Add a cup of boiling water, and while it's steeping for five minutes, carefully lean over and inhale the fumes. Then, strain and drink the liquid. Repeat three to four times a day while sick.

Catch more viruses with vinegar. Like the lemon, vinegar is acidic, and inhaling its fumes makes your respiratory tract a less inviting place for viruses. Mix $\frac{1}{2}$ cup vinegar with $\frac{1}{2}$ cup boiling water in a jar, and inhale the steam (being careful not to burn yourself or get the mixture in your eyes).

Food Poisoning

❖ ❖ ❖ ❖

Mrs. Renfro's potato salad looked so good at the church potluck that you didn't care that it probably should have been on ice. It tasted okay at the time, so why the cramps and sudden stomach pain? Food safety sits on a line as thin as a guitar string: One step over the edge, and you're in for a nasty case of food poisoning.

Food poisoning is rarely life-threatening; in fact, it usually runs its course in 24 hours. However, once it's started, it's like a runaway train—you're not going to stop it. The following commonsense tips, however, may help minimize your discomfort.

Practice prevention. The best way to treat food poisoning is to avoid getting it in the first place. You can take several precautions at home by following these tips:

✿ Refrigerate mixed foods, such as salads with mayonnaise and foods that contain dairy products.

✿ Thaw meat in the refrigerator, not at room temperature.

✿ Stuff turkeys or roasts just before cooking—or cook the stuffing separately.

✿ Keep perishable foods cold.

✿ Cook meat thoroughly—whole beef, lamb, and veal should be cooked to at least 145 degrees Fahrenheit (for medium-rare); ground beef, lamb, pork, and veal, as well as whole pork, should be cooked to at least 160 degrees Fahrenheit; and whole poultry (or thighs and wings individually) should be cooked to 180 degrees Fahrenheit (breasts should be cooked to 170 degrees Fahrenheit; ground poultry is okay at 165 degrees Fahrenheit).

✿ Wash hands, utensils, and surfaces with soap and very hot water after handling meat or eggs.

Replace your body's fluids. You need to keep drinking non-alcoholic and noncaffeinated liquids to avoid dehydration, especially if you have diarrhea. Decaffeinated soda, decaffeinated tea with sugar, and water are your best bets, but even eating gelatin will help.

There's more to gain with plain. When your stomach is flopping around like a fish out of water, you shouldn't touch fatty or highly seasoned foods. If you feel you can eat, go with clear liquids, plain toast, mashed potatoes, bananas, or other bland foods.

Let it flow. Vomiting and experiencing diarrhea are like cleaning the gutters: They're dirty jobs, but if you don't do them, you're going to be stuck with a whole bunch of debris you don't want. Your body is trying to expel what's making you feel bad, and you need to trust its self-healing powers. Don't take over-the-counter antidiarrheal or antinausea drugs; they'll only interfere with your body's own defenses.

Warm up a bit. A warm, but not too hot, hot-water bottle placed on the abdomen may help ease the pain of cramps.

Pump in potassium. Vomiting and diarrhea can deplete your body's supply of potassium, a mineral the body needs to perform a variety of functions, including keeping your heart beating. In fact, an extreme potassium imbalance can even be fatal. Start replenishing your potassium about a day after the symptoms first hit by drinking sports drinks or eating a banana or two.

Headaches

❖ ❖ ❖ ❖

No, someone isn't standing behind you clanging a cowbell—it just feels that way. Headaches debilitate from the top down—if your head is pounding, you don't want to do anything else. If you get hit with frequent, severe headaches several times a month, or if your headaches last a couple of days, you need to see your doctor. The same goes for headaches that come on with physical exertion or are accompanied by changes in vision, weakness, numbness, or limb paralysis. But if your skull only smarts on occasion, don't automatically reach for pain pills. Try these tips first:

Go dark. Resting in a dark room is a great way to relieve a headache, especially if your symptoms resemble those of a migraine (such as

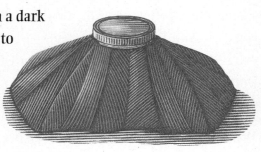

severe pain on one side of the head, nausea, blurred vision, and extreme sensitivity to light). Bright light may also cause headaches, so try wearing sunglasses when outside.

Ice it. Cover your eyes with a washcloth dipped in ice-cold water or place an ice pack on the pain site. For most people, using ice as soon as possible after the onset of the headache will relieve the pain within 20 minutes.

Or, bring the heat. If you're cold to the idea of ice, try putting a warm washcloth over your eyes or on the site of the pain. Leave the compress on for half an hour, rewarming it as necessary.

Cut down on caffeine. We love caffeine because it perks us up; however, it also tenses our muscles and increases anxiety, and both situations trigger headaches. Consuming too much caffeine can also cause headache-inducing insomnia. Try slowly cutting back on caffeine until you're drinking only about 150 milligrams per day (the equivalent of one five-ounce cup of coffee).

Was It Something You Ate?

Eating particular foods can cause headaches in some folks. Be on the lookout for certain ingredients that are well-known headache triggers:

Tyramine and other amines. Tyramine is an amino acid known to promote headaches, nausea, and high blood pressure in certain individuals. A wide variety of vittles harbor tyramine, including aged cheeses, processed meats, peanuts, broad beans, lentils, avocados, bananas, fresh-baked bread, red wine and other alcoholic beverages, and pickled foods. A related headache-causing amine is phenylalanine, which is found in chocolate, among other foods. Even citrus fruits contain an amine that triggers headaches in some people.

Monosodium glutamate (MSG). This purported flavor enhancer is also found in a wide variety of foods, although it is not always clearly identified on food labels (ask your doctor or a dietitian which other words you should look for). It is most commonly found in Chinese food, canned food, soup, soy sauce, seasonings and tenderizers, and processed meat.

Nitrates and nitrites. These preservatives are often added to luncheon and other processed meats, such as bologna, salami, hot dogs, bacon, ham, and smoked fish.

Sleep like a farmer. Farmers' lives are regimented by schedules that must be kept, so they wake up and go to sleep at about the same time every day. Why is this important for you if you don't have to milk cows or slop hogs? Oversleeping can create changes in body chemistry that set off migraines and other headaches. Going to bed and getting up at the same time every day—including weekends—keeps your body in a stable rhythm.

Make a mint. Many
North American
Indian tribes used
peppermint and
spearmint as head-
ache remedies because

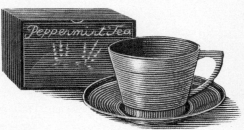

the mints have anti-inflammatory proper-
ties. Put one ounce of dried mint leaves in a one-quart jar
and fill with boiling water. Cover tightly to prevent the
escape of the aromatic constituents. Drink $\frac{1}{2}$ cup of the tea
two to four times a day.

Ask rosemary and sage for help. Another folk remedy for
headache pain is a tea of rosemary and sage. Between them,
these two herbs have 20 anti-inflammatory properties,
most notably rosmarinic acid, which acts similarly to aspirin. (Do not ingest rosemary in any amount exceeding those
usually found in foods, because such large doses may cause
side effects including stomach irritation, kidney damage,
seizures, increased menstrual bleeding, and miscarriage.)

Put one teaspoon of crushed rosemary leaves and one teaspoon of crushed sage leaves in a cup, and fill the cup with
boiling water. Cover the cup well to prevent the helpful
substances from escaping. Let steep until the tea reaches room
temperature, then drink $\frac{1}{2}$ cup two to three times a day for
two or three days.

Heartburn

That big Sunday supper of fried chicken, mashed potatoes and gravy, green bean casserole, fried okra, and apple pie sure hit the spot. But it's been four hours, and now it feels like someone lit a brush fire in your chest. You didn't eat anything spicy, so why the heartburn?

The truth is heartburn isn't all about spicy food. It isn't even about your heart. The burn comes when the industrial-strength acids your stomach releases to digest food slip up into the esophagus in a process called acid reflux. Frequent exposure to acid can damage the esophagus, making it difficult for food to pass. In extreme cases, acid reflux can lead to cancer of the esophagus. This is obviously serious business, so if the following simple tips don't put out your fire, talk with your doc.

Keep your head up. You can protect your esophagus while you sleep by raising the head of your bed. That way, gravity helps keep your stomach contents where they belong. Put wooden blocks under the legs at the head of your bed to raise it about six inches.

Stay up. The couch is not your friend after you eat a meal. People with a full stomach who lie down are asking for trouble. Wait at least an hour before you recline.

Avoid bedtime snacks. It's best if you can wait two to three hours—the time it takes the stomach to empty—after eating before you go to bed.

Pass on seconds. A full stomach may partly empty in the wrong direction.

Loosen your belt. Tight clothing can push on your stomach and contribute to reflux.

Lose the fat. Abdominal fat pressing against the stomach can force the contents back up. Besides, exercise is the best thing you can do for your health.

Eat right. High-fat and fried foods take longer to digest, and if they're in your stomach longer, the odds are better that digestive juices will come back up. It's best to avoid these foods if you have heartburn trouble. Spicy foods and black pepper cause trouble for some people, too. Instead, go farm-fresh and minimally processed—fresh fruits and vegetables, lean meats, fat-free dairy, and complex carbohydrates are better choices. Fruits, vegetables, and complex carbohydrates are high in fiber, which acts like nature's broom, keeping things moving through your digestive tract and preventing the system from backing up (or reversing course).

Don't smoke. Nicotine from cigarette smoke irritates the valve that normally prevents the stomach contents from rising back up into the esophagus. So smokers tend to get heartburn more often.

Cut down on coffee. There are conflicting data, but according to some studies, the caffeine in coffee relaxes the valve that's meant to keep stomach acid from sloshing up into your esophagus. But the oils in the coffee beans may play a role in the problem as well, because even decaffeinated coffee has been shown in some studies to cause acid reflux. Experiment yourself to see if cutting your coffee intake or switching to decaf lessens your heartburn.

Insomnia

❖ ❖ ❖ ❖

Country folks who live in quiet, wide-open spaces aren't immune to insomnia, the chronic inability to get quality sleep. Whether you wake to a screaming alarm clock or a crowing rooster, there is no more frustrating sound when you haven't been able to get any good shut-eye. The American Academy of Sleep Medicine says adults need seven to eight hours of sleep a night, but almost a third of us say we get less than six hours. Obviously, we're not sleeping as well as we should be, no matter where we live.

Insomnia is one of the least-understood sleep disorders. Still, experts have come up with some simple strategies you can try to help improve the quality and increase the amount of sleep you get. Most authorities agree that you should only try pharmaceutical sleep aids under a doctor's care because the pills come with serious warnings.

Get up. Don't lie in bed tossing and turning. If you can't fall asleep after 15 to 20 minutes, get up and do a quiet, low-key activity, such as reading or listening to relaxing music. Then, hit the sack and try again.

But also stay in your bed. Switching beds or moving to the couch will likely only leave you feeling unsettled. Learn to associate sleep with your bed only.

Say no to naps. It's best to let yourself get good and sleepy during the day so it will be easier to get to sleep at night.

Improve your bunk. Catching your Z's is harder if you don't have a comfortable bed. Be sure your mattress and pillows aren't too hard or soft, your blankets aren't too heavy, and your sheets aren't tucked in too tightly.

Alcohol isn't the answer. Although alcohol may help you fall asleep, it is also likely to wake you up during the night by producing a headache, stomachache, or full bladder. And once alcohol's sedative effect wears off, there's a rebound effect that can actually keep you up.

Limit caffeine. Cap your coffee at two cups a day. And stay away from the stimulating stuff, in either food or beverages, after noon.

Stay on schedule. Going to bed and waking at the same times, even on the weekends, is very important. If you can't sleep one night, get up at your usual time the next morning and don't take any naps. You'll probably be out like a light come bedtime the next night.

Take a hot bath. Hot water can relax the muscles and ease the mind, so taking a hot bath an hour or two before bedtime is a great way to wind down and get ready for sleep.

Some folks add the aromas of soothing herbs, like valerian, hop, chamomile, or lavendar. Cover one ounce of your chosen herb with a quart of boiling water, let steep for a couple of minutes, strain out the herbs, and add the herb water to your bath.

Drink warm milk. Some people find it soothing, but the effect may be more psychological than physical. Milk does contain small amounts of the hormone melatonin and the amino acid tryptophan, both of which promote sleep, but research hasn't proved there is enough of either to knock you out. You'll want to avoid this strategy if you wake frequently to urinate.

Don't go to bed hungry. If your tummy is grumbling for food, have a light snack before you hit the sack.

Try some tea. Many people find decaffeinated herbal tea, particularly chamomile tea, good for sleep. Check your grocer's shelves.

Motion Sickness
❖ ❖ ❖ ❖

The history of motion sickness has to stretch back years in America. There's no way pioneers traveled hundreds of miles in covered wagons over bumpy terrain and didn't get hit by sweating, light-headedness, hyperventilation, nausea, and vomiting. Modern transportation hasn't eliminated motion sickness (an affliction caused when the eyes and inner ears send conflicting sensory information to the brain). It can strike in a pickup, train, boat, plane—even in a movie theater when you're watching motion on the big screen.

However, you don't have to reach for medication to ward off that queasiness before you take to the road, skies, or seas. There are simple ways to outsmart the mechanism behind motion sickness. Try the following:

Pick the right seat. To get the smoothest ride, sit in the front seat of a car, an aisle seat over a wing on a plane, a car toward the front on a train, or a cabin toward the center of a ship.

And stay seated. Being tossed around isn't going to keep your stomach settled.

Face forward. Face the direction you are traveling, so the forward motion your body feels will match the signals your eyes send to your brain.

Steady your head. Avoid moving your head suddenly, because this can aggravate motion sickness.

Look off into the distance. Focus on a steady point away from the rocking boat, plane, or car. If there isn't a tree, barn, or something else in the distance to focus on, stare out at the horizon, where the sky meets the earth (or water). This allows your eyes to see that you are moving without making you dizzy.

Don't read in the car. Reading focuses your eyes on a stationary object while your body feels the motion of the moving vehicle. This creates that sensory contradiction that causes motion sickness.

Avoid heavy foods and odors. The smell of spicy or greasy foods and strong odors can prompt motion sickness before or during a trip. So skip the stop at the roadside diner and don't choose the plane or train seat next to the guy eating the fried chicken.

Say no to alcohol. Avoid alcoholic beverages before and during a trip. Booze can worsen motion sickness.

Stay away from the sick. Let someone with a sturdier stomach tend to the sick, especially if you're prone to turn the color of a John Deere tractor when you're around the queasy.

Travel with ginger ale. Ginger is used to comfort all kinds of stomach woes, so try sipping a bit of ginger ale (containing real ginger) if your stomach is taking its own trip.

Muscle Pain

❖ ❖ ❖ ❖

Hard work sometimes comes with a little pain. Whether you're pitchin' hay, diggin' fencepost holes, or just helping a friend move, you're probably going to end up with some muscle pain—but the work still has to get done.

Overworked muscles hurt because the muscle fibers actually break down. This is especially true with muscles that aren't used on a regular basis. The muscles also swell slightly, and by-products of muscle breakdown accumulate. All this makes you stiff and sore. Of course, a muscle can also cramp. A cramp is a spasm caused by anything that interferes with the contraction and relaxation of the muscle. The tight contraction of the muscle restricts the blood flow to the area, causing the intense pain.

Muscle soreness and muscle cramps generally aren't life-threatening, but they can keep you from work—and play. Try these tips before popping any aspirin or ibuprofen.

Cool off. If you know you've overworked your muscles, hop in a cold shower or a cold bath to help prevent or minimize inflammation and soreness. You can also apply ice packs to the muscles for 20 to 30 minutes every hour for 24 to 72 hours after the activity. Cold constricts the blood vessels, which reduces blood flow and thus inflammation in the area.

Avoid heat. Heat is the wrong first step for treating sore muscles, because it dilates blood vessels and increases circulation to the area, which in turn leads to more swelling, and more soreness and stiffness. It takes about three or four days for the swelling and soreness to diminish; after that, you can take hot baths to help relax the muscles.

Pitch the sports creams. Those topical "sports" creams don't do much beyond causing a chemical reaction that leaves your skin (but not the underlying muscles) feeling warm or cold. Save your money and apply ice instead.

Do easy stretches. You don't want to move when you're sore and stiff, but stretching those muscles can actually help ease your discomfort. Go easy, though, and warm up first with a 20-minute walk.

Take a swim. Hit the swimming hole of your choice to remedy those sore muscles. The cold water helps reduce inflammation, and moving muscles in water helps stretch them out and ease soreness.

Stop. If you get a muscle cramp while working or exercising, stop what you're doing. Trying to "work through" a cramp might cause more damage.

Drink plenty of fluids. Dehydration can cause acute cramps, especially when you're working hard or exercising for an hour or longer when it's hot. Stay hydrated, preferably with water, before, during, and after your activity.

Stretch and squeeze a cramp. Stretch a cramped-up muscle while gently kneading and squeezing it at the point of tightness (you'll be able to feel a knot or a hard bulge of muscle). Try to feel which way the muscle has contracted, and stretch it in the opposite direction.

Adjust your diet. A potassium deficiency can sometimes cause muscle cramps, so try adding potassium-rich foods to your plate. These include apricots, avocados, bananas, beans, meat (including poultry and fish), potatoes, spinach, and tomatoes.

Wrap up. Warm muscles are less likely to cramp up, so dress in warm layers when you're working or exercising outside in cold weather.

Walk it out. If you do work out a cramp, don't jump back into your activity whole hog. Ease back into things by walking slowly for a few minutes to get the blood flowing back to the muscles.

Nausea and Vomiting

O ne minute you're sitting on the porch, enjoying a nice relaxing chat with the neighbor. The next, you're bolting from your seat like a spooked horse, in search of the nearest bathroom. You're never ready for nausea and vomiting to strike because they can come on so quickly. Whether caused by a virus, bacterium, or some other condition, it's never fun when your settled stomach suddenly feels like it's riding the Whirly Bird at the county fair.

The good news is that nausea and vomiting usually pass quickly. But if vomiting is violent, if it lasts for more than a day, or if the vomited material contains blood or looks like coffee grounds, see a doctor right away. Otherwise try the following advice:

Hunker down. The best thing to do when your stomach is doing flips is rest. It will leave your body with more energy to fight off an invader or eject an offending substance.

Herbs & Spices for a Happier Stomach

Nature can provide some relief for nausea and, if necessary, for vomiting, although it's usually best to let vomiting run its course. Check your pantry for the following natural stomach soothers (if you're pregnant or if you have a chronic health problem, ask your doctor before trying any of these remedies):

Cinnamon. Put ½ teaspoon of cinnamon powder in a cup, and fill the cup with boiling water. Cover, let steep five minutes, then sip.

Ginger. Put ½ teaspoon of powdered ginger spice in a cup, and fill the cup with boiling water. Cover, let steep ten minutes, then sip.

Peppermint. Drop one tablespoon of mint leaves in a one-pint jar, and fill the jar with boiling water. Let stand 20 to 30 minutes, shaking the bottle from time to time to mix the contents. Strain out the leaves, then sip.

Let it flow. If you can, try to resist the urge to take over-the-counter or even natural medicine to stop vomiting, at least at the start, because vomiting is your body's way of getting rid of something that doesn't belong.

Stick to clear liquids. An upset stomach doesn't need the extra work of digesting food. Stick to fluids until you feel better and have stopped vomiting. Clear, room-temperature liquids, such as water or diluted noncitrus fruit juices, are easier to digest, and they also prevent dehydration.

Clean livin' works wonders. Alcohol can be very irritating to the stomach. If you already have an upset stomach, now is certainly not the time to tip a few. And if you got sick after drinking, forget about the "hair of the dog that bit you," unless you want a pit bull running around in your gut. You should also steer clear of fatty foods, highly seasoned foods, caffeinated drinks, and cigarettes.

Eat easy-to-digest foods. When you're ready to belly back up to the table, choose soft, plain foods, such as bread, unbuttered toast, steamed fish, and bananas, but stay away from high-fiber foods. Another tip is to start with small amounts of food and slowly build up to full meals.

Poison Ivy, Oak, and Sumac

C ountry folks are closer to the land than most people, but there is such a thing as being too close. That's the case when it comes to poison ivy, oak, and sumac, three plants whose oils cause an itchy rash in about 85 percent of the U.S. population. Unless you're in Alaska, Hawaii, or certain parts of the Nevada desert, one of these weeds is just waiting to make you miserable. All three produce similar reactions, so if you're allergic to one, you'd best avoid the other two as well.

The offending oils start penetrating the skin within minutes of contact. Within 12 to 48 hours, a red, itchy rash appears, followed by blisters that may weep and then get crusty. The rash will clear up after about ten days. If you're very sensitive to the oils, your skin will swell up, the rash can be severe and painful, and the reaction may take up to three weeks to clear if left untreated. See a doctor right away if you are highly sensitive to these plants and you come into contact with one of them. For everyone else, heed the following advice (although many tips refer to poison ivy, they should work for poison oak and poison sumac, too).

Prevent the Rash

You're always better off avoiding a rash than treating it, so use these prevention tips.

Don't leaf it to chance. Know what the poisonous plants in your area look like, because appearance will vary, even within a state. Poison ivy is found east of the Rockies, poison oak grows in the West and Southwest, and poison sumac thrives east of the Mississippi River.

Typically, poison ivy is a vine or a low shrub with grayish white berries and smooth, pointed leaves that are usually clustered in groups of three. The reddish leaves turn green in the summer and redden again by autumn. Poison oak is a shrub or small tree with greenish-white berries and oaklike leaves that also usually appear in groups of three. Poison sumac is a woody shrub with smooth-edged leaves and cream-colored berries that is found in swampy, boggy areas. Your local cooperative extension office might be able to give you details about what grows in your area.

Cover up. Long pants, long-sleeved shirts, boots, and gloves provide a barrier between you and the plant's oils.

Keep your pets out of the woods. If you get a rash from poison ivy but you haven't been near any plants, you might have your pet to thank, because poison ivy oils can cling to the animal's fur. Petting the critter then transfers the oils to you.

Rinse your clothes outside. If you think you've brushed against some poison ivy, the oil may be all over your clothes. If you wear those clothes inside, you might transfer the oil to rugs or furniture. Water deactivates the oil, so rinse off everything—including shoes and camping and hunting gear—before you head in.

Get wet—fast. If poison ivy has touched your skin, rinse off right away. If you can get to water within five to ten minutes after contact with the plant, you may be able to wash off the oil before all of it sinks in.

Use rubbing alcohol. Rubbing alcohol might extract some oil from the skin because the oil sinks in gradually. Pour rubbing alcohol on the exposed areas and then rinse well with water. Don't use an alcohol wipe or a cloth soaked in alcohol, because it can transfer the oil somewhere else.

Treat the Rash

If you weren't lucky enough to avoid poison ivy, the rash doesn't have to be that bad.

Cool the itch. A cool bath may help ease the itch. Another option is to place cold compresses on the rash for a few minutes every hour.

Call on calamine. Calamine lotion can be soothing and may help dry the rash. Don't slather on too much, though, because the pink stuff can seal the pores.

Soak in oats or soda. Bathing in cool or lukewarm water mixed with oatmeal or baking soda can help dry out oozing blisters and help soothe irritated skin.

Psoriasis

❖ ❖ ❖ ❖

Psoriasis is a noncontagious, chronic skin condition that produces plaques—which are round, dry, scaly patches of varying size that are covered with white, gray, or silvery-white scales. Although there are several other types of psoriasis, this plaque-forming variety (called plaque psoriasis) is the most common.

Doctors aren't sure what causes psoriasis, but it tends to run in families. Most experts agree that it is an autoimmune condition, meaning the body attacks its own healthy cells. The body accelerates the growth and turnover of skin cells, which produces the itchy plaques. Psoriasis can be mild one day and severe the next. Treatment is difficult, because what works for one person may not work for another, and treatments that were once effective for an individual often become ineffective. Although psoriasis has no cure, it can be managed.

Moisturize. Moisturizing battles dry skin, reduces inflammation, helps keep the skin flexible, and makes plaque

Kitchen Help

You can make anti-itch remedies with fixins from your kitchen. The National Psoriasis Foundation suggests the following recipes:

❖ Dissolve $1\frac{1}{2}$ cups baking soda in three gallons water to use in an anti-itch compress.

❖ Add a handful of Epsom salts to your bathwater.

❖ Add two teaspoons olive oil to a large glass of milk for a soothing bath oil (but use extra caution to avoid slipping when getting into and out of the tub).

❖ Toss a cup of oats in your bathwater, or add a commercial bath product that contains "colloidal oats."

scales less noticeable. The heaviest, or greasiest, lotions work best, but cheaper household alternatives, like cooking oils, lard, or petroleum jelly, work well, too.

Get some rays. Most folks aren't advised to spend time out in the sun, but the sun's ultraviolet (UV) light often causes psoriasis to clear up (even though the reasons why it works aren't clear). You shouldn't act like a snake on a highway, though, because a sunburn can cause the disease to flare.

The National Psoriasis Foundation suggests applying a thin layer of mineral oil to affected areas of skin. This will keep the skin moist and magnify the sun's effects. But because mineral oil also makes you more likely to get burned, stay out for only short periods of time. You should also apply sunscreen (with a sun protection factor of at least 15) on the skin that isn't affected by psoriasis.

Get wet. Swim, shower, jump in the tub, or apply wet compresses; any way to get your skin wet helps because water rehydrates the skin and can help soften and remove thick psoriasis scales. Regular soaking also helps reduce itching and redness of lesions. Don't make the water too hot, though, because that will actually increase itching. And be sure to slather on that thick lotion immediately afterward to lock in moisture.

Reach for vinegar. Vinegar has been used for thousands of years to soothe burns and inflammation. Vinegar is also a disinfectant. Try adding apple cider vinegar to your bath or dab it directly on your skin with a cotton ball.

Snoring

❖ ❖ ❖ ❖

If sleeping next to you reminds your bedmate of a 2 A.M. freight train or an old diesel tractor in need of a tune-up, you're probably used to some strained mornings. But snoring doesn't just strain your relationships; it can also strain your breathing. This is especially true with sleep apnea, a dangerous condition that causes a person to stop breathing during sleep. It has also been linked to cardiovascular disease. If you're among the one-third of adults who snore, read on for tips that will help you and your sleep partner get better sack time.

Sleep on your side. You're more likely to snore if you're lying on your back, and sleeping on your stomach is stressful on your neck.

Quiet the racket with tennis balls. No, you're not going to sleep with them in your mouth, you're going to use them to keep you from rolling onto your back during sleep. Sew a long, tight pocket onto the back of your pajama top, and put two or three tennis balls into it. If you don't sew, shove the tennis balls in a sock and pin the sock to the back of your pajama top.

Avoid alcohol and tranquilizers. Alcohol and sleeping pills can depress your central nervous system and relax the muscles of your throat and jaw, making snoring more likely.

Lighten your load. Excess body weight, especially around the neck, puts pressure on the airway, causing it to partially collapse. The tissues then vibrate as air passes through the constricted airway, causing your snoring.

Stop smoking. Smoking damages the respiratory system because smoke irritates and inflames airway tissues. The inflammation causes the airway to narrow.

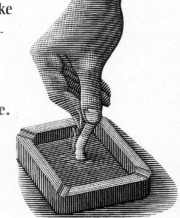

Stay on your shut-eye schedule. You're more likely to snore if you're exhausted, so get plenty of sleep. Go to bed and get up at the same time each day to help prevent problems.

See a doctor if you are pregnant and snoring. Pregnant women might start snoring because of weight gain or because hormonal changes cause muscles to relax. Whatever the case, snoring during pregnancy may rob your baby of oxygen, so talk with your doctor about it.

Rise up. Raising your head can take pressure off the airway and make breathing easier. But don't just prop up your head, because a bent neck can inhibit breathing and cause neck pain. Instead, raise the head of the bed by putting blocks under the bedposts, or prop up your upper body with pillows.

Sore Throat

❖ ❖ ❖ ❖

Most sore throats are minor and caused by simple problems (a cold or a stuffy nose, for instance), but try believing that when it feels like someone is scraping their spurs down your gullet every time you swallow. We've rounded up some tips for minor sore throats that come with colds or allergies. If you have a severe sore throat that lasts two or three days, or one that is accompanied by a fever, body aches and pains, and malaise, you might have strep throat, a potentially serious bacterial infection. See your doctor if you have these symptoms.

Salt your wound. Make a saline solution by adding half a teaspoon of salt to a cup of very warm water, and gargle with it. The salt water draws water out of inflamed tissue, which relieves swelling and makes it difficult for the offending bacteria and viruses to survive.

Line up some Listerine. It's not tasty, but bacteria don't get much hospitality from Listerine mouthwash. Pour a small amount into a cup and gargle it a couple of times a day.

Sip hot liquids. Drinking hot fluids, such as coffee, tea, or hot lemonade, coats the tissue in your throat and has benefits similar to applying hot packs to infected skin.

Kick back with some candy. As with any ailment, putting your feet up and relaxing goes a long way toward helping you feel better. That's because taking it easy leaves your body more energy to fight the infection. And while you're resting, suck on some hard candy. Some doctors say sugar can help soothe a sore throat and ease the ticklish cough that may come with it. Sucking on hard candy—even the sugar-free kind—also keeps your mouth and throat moist, which will make you feel more comfortable.

Get under a tent. No, you're not going camping, you're getting under a steam tent. Carefully put your face over a bowl of steaming hot water and cover your head with a towel to keep the steam in. The steam soothes dry, raw tissue and helps open your constricted airway.

Keep drinking. Drink as much nonalcoholic fluid as you can—at least eight to ten 8-ounce glasses throughout the day. If your throat is well lubricated, you'll be more comfortable, and staying hydrated may help your body kick out the infection faster.

Try this tonic. The following recipe came from a book of home remedies that is almost 150 years old, and some doctors say it still works wonders. (Do not give it, or anything else that contains honey, to children younger than two because honey can cause infant botulism and allergic reactions in youngsters.)

Mix one tablespoon of honey and one tablespoon of apple cider vinegar with eight ounces of hot water. Sip this mixture slowly, but don't let it get cold. You can use this as often as you desire.

Open up to onion syrup. It won't be anyone's first choice to cover their flapjacks, but onion syrup is full of antimicrobial substances that attack infecting organisms like the one that might be making your throat sore. (These same antimicrobial substances are also what make onions stink and make your eyes water when you're cutting them.)

Slice a raw onion, put it in a bowl or baking pan, and then cover the onion slices with sugar. Allow the onion to sit at room temperature until syrup forms (you don't need to add water because the sugar sucks the juice out of the onion). It may take a day or two for the syrup to form this way, but you can speed up the process by putting the sugar-covered onions in the oven and baking them at a medium heat until the syrup forms. Take a tablespoon of syrup as needed.

Stings

❖ ❖ ❖ ❖

Those who live in the country know the occasional sting from a bee, yellow jacket, hornet, wasp, fire ant, or other stinging critter is all part of the business of being outside. After all, insects have a job to do, too. For millions of people who are allergic to stinging insects, though, a sting can mean more than a little pain and swelling—it can mean a trip to the hospital because of sudden hives, wheezing, difficulty breathing, dizziness, and nausea. In the most severe type of allergic reaction (called anaphylaxis), shock, unconsciousness, and cardiac arrest can occur.

For most people, however, a sting is little more than a minor nuisance. And it's one you can do something about.

Ease the Pain

Try these simple suggestions for relieving pain caused by a sting, but keep an eye out for signs of a more severe reaction so you can get medical help immediately, if necessary.

Tender some relief. The same product that makes cheap cuts of meat more palatable can do wonders for a sting. As soon as you feel the insect's wrath, mix a few drops of water with a teaspoon of unseasoned meat tenderizer and apply it to the sting site. An enzyme in the tenderizer, either papain or bromelain, dissolves the toxins injected by the insect. If you're exploring in an area where stinging insects live, carry a bottle filled with the premixed solution.

This remedy only works if used immediately after you're stung. You can't wait too long, or the venom proteins will penetrate too deeply into your skin and be out of reach of the papain or bromelain.

Use baking soda as a backup. If you don't have any meat tenderizer, you can make a paste of baking soda and water and apply it to the sting site. Baking soda doesn't neutralize insect venom, but it will help ease itching and swelling.

Take out the stinger. Bees and some yellow jackets have barbed stingers that stay in your skin after the insect attacks. (Other stinging insects have smooth stingers that remain intact on the bug.) That stinger will continue to release venom for several minutes unless you get it out. However, you don't want to squeeze, grab, or press the stinger, because that will pump even more venom into your skin. Use a clean knife blade, or even a fingernail, to gently scrape the stinger out.

Go cold. If you can't do anything else, go with the old standby—ice. Rubbing ice over the sting site can help with pain because it reduces inflammation and swelling, but ice won't neutralize the toxins.

Favor some flavor. Both garlic and onions contain broad-spectrum antibiotic and anti-inflammatory substances that can disinfect and soothe a bite or sting. Crush a clove of garlic and mix it with a little water, then apply the paste directly to the sting area. Place a thick slice of onion over the area, and leave it on as long as you like (or as long as folks can stand to be around you).

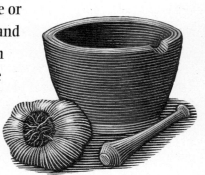

Prevent Future Stings

An ounce of prevention really is worth a pound of cure when it comes to insect stings, even when the insects themselves weigh much less than an ounce. Try the following to keep yourself from being stung in the first place.

Make your sweat unappealing. Some bug brainiacs think insects like certain varieties of sweat or body odor more than others. According to one theory, changing how your sweat smells may keep away insects. Believers in this theory suggest adding extra garlic and onions to your vittles. The downside, though, is that you might repel people, too.

Watch what you wear. Bright, flowery clothes and rough fabrics are attractive to insects for some reason. When you know you're going to be outside, wear smooth fabric and light-colored outfits that are white, tan, green, or khaki.

Go fragrance-free. Bugs also like fancy-smelling people. Perfume and cologne, as well as scented aftershave, hair spray, and soap, will attract insects. Try going natural to avoid those painful stings.

Keep your shoes on. Bees are attracted to ground clover, and yellow jacket nests are in the ground, so going shoeless can mean stepping into trouble.

Sunburn Pain

❖ ❖ ❖

Those who live in rural areas often do hard work outside, especially in the summer, when the sun beats down and there isn't an air conditioner in sight. So why is it that tank tops and shorts aren't standard country attire?

These folks understand that outside work is hard on the body, what with the bugs and critters and flying debris and sharp tools. They also understand the wisdom of covering skin as much as possible to prevent sunburn during long days outdoors. But the sun still gets the best of them on occasion, too, so they often turn to traditional country remedies, like those that follow, to cope. Of course, even the best sunburn treatment can't undo the deeper damage that the sun inflicts on skin, the kind that can lead to skin cancer. The best way to protect skin from pain and permanent damage is to stay out of the sun. And if you do get a sunburn and blisters form, you need to see your doctor right away.

Ease the Pain

Try the following tips next time you're overexposed.

Stay inside. Sunburned skin is extremely vulnerable to additional burning, so stay indoors for a few days. You won't find much protection in the shade, because damaging ultraviolet light still gets through. It also gets through your clothes, so just play it safe inside.

Stay cool. Slip into a tub of chilly water to ease some of the burn's sting. It's best to avoid soap—just let the water put the painful fire out—but don't stay in the tub too long, because an extended bath can dry out the skin. Don't towel off aggressively when you're done, either; just gently pat your skin dry. If you're away from home, you can apply cool compresses to the burn area throughout the day. Soak a washcloth in cool water and apply it directly to the sunburn (but never use ice or an ice pack).

Add to the bath. Putting oatmeal or baking soda in your bathwater may help soothe skin even more than soaking in plain water. Wrap some oatmeal in cheesecloth or some gauze and then hold the bundle under the faucet as the tub fills. If you'd rather use baking soda, just sprinkle it liberally into the water. Stay in the tub only 15 to 20 minutes to avoid drying out your skin.

Moisturize. Whether you use a wet compress or you get in the tub, you need to put on lotion when you're done. You can put the lotion in the refrigerator before you use it to get some extra cooling relief.

Use aloe vera. The aloe vera plant produces gel-like juice that eases the sting of burns and limits skin redness if the gel is applied immediately to a new burn. The plants are easy to grow inside or outside, so if you have a green thumb, you can have soothing relief straight from the soil anytime. Simply slit open one of the broad leaves and apply the gel directly to the burn five or six times per day for several days. If you don't want to grow your own plants, you can buy aloe vera gel at almost any drugstore.

Mix in some vinegar. Try dousing your sunburned skin with a little vinegar several times a day. Vinegar is both astringent and antiseptic, and, like cool water, it helps to prevent blisters. You can dilute the vinegar with water if your skin is very sensitive.

Prevent the Burn

Of course, the best way to avoid the pain of sunburn is to avoid being burned in the first place. You'll also protect your skin from cancer if you limit your exposure to the sun.

Cover your skin. According to the Skin Cancer Foundation, hats and clothing made of dark, tightly woven materials absorb ultraviolet light better than cotton fabrics in lighter shades. In addition, dry fabrics offer more protection than wet ones, so change your shirt if it gets wet.

Set a screen. The Centers for Disease Control and Prevention recommends wearing sunscreen with a sun protection factor (SPF) of at least 15. Apply a thick layer of sunscreen

20 to 30 minutes before
exposure to the sun
to allow the skin
to absorb it.
Reapply the
stuff every two
hours—more often if you're sweating or getting wet. And
don't forget the tops of your ears, your hairline and the area
of your scalp where your hair parts, the "V" of your chest,
your nose, and the tops of your hands and feet. You'll also
want to use a lip balm that has an SPF of at least 15.

Be wary of reflected light. Umbrellas and shade trees provide only moderate protection from ultraviolet light, and
they don't protect you from rays reflected off sand, water,
ice and snow (yes, you can get sunburned in the winter!),
and many other surfaces. Ultraviolet light also penetrates
about a foot into water, so being in a pool, lake, or ocean
doesn't provide much protection.

Watch the clock. The sun's rays are most intense between
10:00 A.M. and 4:00 P.M., so stay indoors or wear plenty of
sunscreen if you're out during this time of day.

Toothache

❖ ❖ ❖ ❖

If you've ever had a toothache, you know that's the one kind of pain that can really make you see red. The stabbing pain or dull throbbing can't seem to get any worse—until you try to eat or drink.

There can be many causes of tooth pain. Perhaps the most common is a minor, momentary twinge that's caused by sensitive teeth. More serious toothaches can be blamed on sinus problems, bruxism (teeth grinding), an issue with the jaw joint, or recent dental work. If it hurts when you bite down, you may have a cavity, a loose filling, a cracked tooth, or damaged pulp (the inner core of the tooth that contains the blood vessels and nerves). Pain that sticks around for more than 30 minutes after eating hot or cold foods can also indicate pulp damage. In general, if a tooth hurts enough to wake you up at night or to interfere with your ability to function normally during the day, see a dentist.

Of course, you can avoid minor toothaches by practicing good dental hygiene, so always follow your dentist's instructions for brushing and flossing. If you do end up with a chopper that smarts like the dickens and it's a Sunday afternoon, you can improvise to get some relief before the dentist's office opens Monday morning.

Call on cloves. Pick up some oil of cloves at your pharmacy and follow the directions for use carefully (too much can lead to poisoning). You'll want to put it only on the tooth and not on the gum, because oil of cloves can burn the senstitive tissues. This remedy isn't a cure; it only temporarily numbs the nerve, but it might help enough until you can see your dentist.

Put it on ice. Holding an ice cube or cold water in your mouth may relieve the pain, but it does aggravate some people's sensitive teeth. If this happens to you, skip the cold stuff.

Keep your head up. Elevating your head can decrease the pressure in the area and ease that throbbing pain.

Rinse. A piece of food that gets stuck in the gum can hurt as much as damaged tooth pulp, so try rinsing your mouth with warm water. Stir one teaspoon of salt in a glass of warm water, swish it around your mouth, then spit it out. Flossing or carefully using a toothpick may do the trick, too.

Go with gum. If exposure to air makes the sore chopper hoppin' mad, you can cover it with a bit of chewed sugarless chewing gum. Use the teeth on the opposite side of the mouth to chew the gum, and only keep it in place until you can get to the dentist.

Warts

❖ ❖ ❖ ❖

Warts are like barn owls—they don't really cause any damage, but they are annoying to have around. Toads aren't to blame for warts, the human papilloma virus

(HPV) is, and the little buggers are contagious. That's why warts can spread like ants at a barbecue.

Common warts are the rough-looking lesions that most often pop up on the hands and fingers. The much smaller, smoother flat warts tend to show up on the hands and on the face. Warts that occur on the soles of the feet are called plantar warts and can sometimes be as large as a quarter. Genital warts, which develop in the genital and anal area, are a whole different ballgame and need a doctor's attention; do not try the following self-help remedies on these.

Before you try any type of treatment, know whether your skin eruption is a wart or another condition. When in doubt, see your doctor. In addition, if you have diabetes, circulation problems, or impaired immunity, do not try any home therapy for wart removal.

Stick to it. Wrap the wart with four layers of adhesive tape, making sure the wrap is snug but not too tight. Leave the tape on for six and a half days, and then remove the tape for half a day. You may need to repeat the procedure for about three to four weeks before the wart disappears. You can try the procedure on a plantar wart, but be sure to use strips of tape that are long enough to be properly secured.

Cast your lot with castor oil. The acid in castor oil probably does the trick by irritating the wart. It works best on small, flat warts that are on the face and on the back of the hands. Apply castor oil to the wart with a cotton swab twice a day.

Warm some water. Soaking plantar warts in very hot water softens the wart and may kill the virus. Be sure the water is not hot enough to cause burns, however.

Keep your shoes on. Warts shed viral particles by the millions, so going shoeless puts you at risk for acquiring a plantar wart. Locker rooms, pools, public or shared showers, even the carpets in hotel rooms harbor a host of germs—not just wart viruses. You can catch any of a number of infections, from scabies to herpes simplex. At the very least, wear a pair of flip-flops.

Stay dry. Warts, especially plantar warts, tend to flourish in a damp environment. As a result, according to the American Academy of Dermatology, people who walk or exercise extensively may be more prone to foot warts. Change your socks any time your feet get sweaty, and use a medicated foot powder to help keep them dry.

Cover your cuts and scrapes. HPV loves finding a good scratch so it can make its way under your skin. By keeping your cuts and scrapes covered, you'll help keep out the wart virus.

Reach for some flavor. Garlic has several antimicrobial properties, and one might work against HPV. Apply petroleum jelly to the healthy skin around the wart to protect the skin from blistering, then apply a small bit of garlic oil extract twice a day for a week or two. You also can try tying or taping a thin slice of garlic to the wart, but studies have shown this isn't as effective as using the oil extract.